THIS TRACKER BELONGS TO

_____

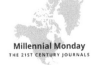

Millennial Monday
THE 21ST CENTURY JOURNALS

Image from rawpixel.com
For more information on the topic we recommend to check: "Atomic Habits: An Easy and Proven Way to Build Good Habits and Break Bad Ones" by James Clear
"The Two Day Rule" by Matt D'Avella on YouTube.com

ABOUT THE 2-DAY RULE HABIT TRACKER

- The 2 Day-Rule tracking system is an amazing tool to build a new habit. And more importantly to transform it into behavior that will be performed automatically later on.

- On the contrary to many "challenge yourself" systems that are very intense and usually short-termed (30 days, 90 days etc.), THE 2-DAY RULE HABIT TRACKER allows for both discipline and schedule to see the results, but is flexible enough to allow your daily life to "happen". The 2-Day Rule tracker helps to keep you motivated and gives sufficient time to take a break as well.

IT IS VERY SIMPLE TO USE:

1. Choose carefully a habit that you would want to have for a long time in your life.

2. Use a calendar in THE 2-DAY RULE TRACKER to check/highlight the days that you implemented the habit. The calendar is undated so you can start any month or week!

3. The only rule: **Don't let yourself take 2 days off in a row for any of your habits. In a week you can take one day off, you can take multiple days off. But not in a row.** For example, if your habit is to work out consistently, never miss 2 consecutive workouts in a row. Life happens, just be sure it doesn't happen 2 days in a row.

THE PSYCHOLOGY UNDERNEATH

- Taking 2 days off makes you to lose the momentum and it is so much easier to skip more days to the point that you lose track completely. We've all been there: any time we would miss a day, often for a good reason, it would trigger a downward spiral. We would feel bad about missing a day, and those bad feelings make it more likely that we'd miss a second day, and then we'd be even more likely to miss a third day.

THE STRUCTURE OF THE TRACKER

- The tracker's minimalistic design makes it easy to use. You'll need less than a minute a day to check the box and see your progress as you stay consistent. The Notes section is optionary to fill in the information about the days that you skipped. In the end of The 2-Day Rule tracker there is a place for extra notes to write your monthly progress and your feelings about the new routine.

- Research shows that when introducing new habits into our life it's better to take it slow and not to take more than 2-3 new habits at a time. THE 2-DAY RULE TRACKER consists of 6 months worth of tracking sheets for 5 different habits.

THIS TRACKER WILL BE WITH YOU ON YOUR JOURNEY TO BUILDING BETTER HABITS AND STRONGER SELF. BEST OF LUCK AND REMEMBER: NEVER SKIP TWICE IN A ROW :)

The Road Is Tough
But the Rider is Tougher.
Good Luck!

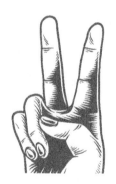

THE 2-DAY RULE TRACKER

_____

HABIT

_____

MONTH

SUN	MON	TUE	WED	THU	FRI	SAT

NOTES

_____

_____

_____

_____

THE 2-DAY RULE TRACKER

HABIT

MONTH

SUN	MON	TUE	WED	THU	FRI	SAT

NOTES

THE 2-DAY RULE TRACKER

_____

HABIT

_____

MONTH

SUN	MON	TUE	WED	THU	FRI	SAT

NOTES

_____

_____

_____

_____

THE 2-DAY RULE TRACKER

HABIT

MONTH

SUN	MON	TUE	WED	THU	FRI	SAT

NOTES

THE 2-DAY RULE TRACKER

HABIT

MONTH

SUN	MON	TUE	WED	THU	FRI	SAT

NOTES

The best time to plant a tree

was 20 years ago.

The second best time

is now.

Chinese Proverb

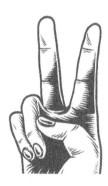

THE 2-DAY RULE TRACKER

_____

HABIT

_____

MONTH

SUN	MON	TUE	WED	THU	FRI	SAT

NOTES

_____

_____

_____

_____

THE 2-DAY RULE TRACKER

_____

HABIT

_____

MONTH

SUN	MON	TUE	WED	THU	FRI	SAT

NOTES

THE 2-DAY RULE TRACKER

_____

HABIT

_____

MONTH

SUN	MON	TUE	WED	THU	FRI	SAT

NOTES

_____

_____

_____

_____

THE 2-DAY RULE TRACKER

_____

HABIT

_____

MONTH

SUN	MON	TUE	WED	THU	FRI	SAT

NOTES

_____

_____

_____

THE 2-DAY RULE TRACKER

HABIT

MONTH

SUN	MON	TUE	WED	THU	FRI	SAT

NOTES

It is better to conquer yourself

than to win a thousand battles.

Then the victory is yours.

It cannot be taken from you.

Not by angels or by demons, heaven or hell.

Buddha

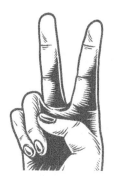

THE 2-DAY RULE TRACKER

_____

HABIT

_____

MONTH

SUN	MON	TUE	WED	THU	FRI	SAT

NOTES

_____

_____

_____

_____

THE 2-DAY RULE TRACKER

HABIT

MONTH

SUN	MON	TUE	WED	THU	FRI	SAT

NOTES

THE 2-DAY RULE TRACKER

_____

HABIT

_____

MONTH

SUN	MON	TUE	WED	THU	FRI	SAT

NOTES

_____

_____

_____

_____

THE 2-DAY RULE TRACKER

HABIT

MONTH

SUN	MON	TUE	WED	THU	FRI	SAT

NOTES

THE 2-DAY RULE TRACKER

_____

HABIT

_____

MONTH

SUN	MON	TUE	WED	THU	FRI	SAT

NOTES

_____

_____

_____

_____

Be not afraid

of growing slowly,

be afraid only

of standing still.

Chinese Proverb

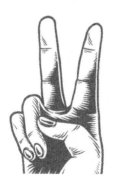

THE 2-DAY RULE TRACKER

_____

HABIT

_____

MONTH

SUN	MON	TUE	WED	THU	FRI	SAT

NOTES

_____

_____

_____

_____

THE 2-DAY RULE TRACKER

_____

HABIT

_____

MONTH

SUN	MON	TUE	WED	THU	FRI	SAT

NOTES

_____

_____

_____

_____

THE 2-DAY RULE TRACKER

_____

HABIT

_____

MONTH

SUN	MON	TUE	WED	THU	FRI	SAT

NOTES
_____

_____

_____

_____

THE 2-DAY RULE TRACKER

HABIT

MONTH

SUN	MON	TUE	WED	THU	FRI	SAT

NOTES

THE 2-DAY RULE TRACKER

_____

HABIT

_____

MONTH

SUN	MON	TUE	WED	THU	FRI	SAT

NOTES

_____

_____

_____

_____

Rule your mind

Or it will rule you

Horace

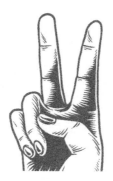

THE 2-DAY RULE TRACKER

_____

HABIT

_____

MONTH

SUN	MON	TUE	WED	THU	FRI	SAT

NOTES

_____

_____

_____

_____

THE 2-DAY RULE TRACKER

_____

HABIT

_____

MONTH

SUN	MON	TUE	WED	THU	FRI	SAT

NOTES

_____

_____

_____

_____

THE 2-DAY RULE TRACKER

_____
HABIT

_____
MONTH

SUN	MON	TUE	WED	THU	FRI	SAT

NOTES
_____
_____
_____
_____

THE 2-DAY RULE TRACKER

HABIT

MONTH

SUN	MON	TUE	WED	THU	FRI	SAT

NOTES

THE 2-DAY RULE TRACKER

_____

HABIT

_____

MONTH

SUN	MON	TUE	WED	THU	FRI	SAT

NOTES
_____
_____
_____
_____

Through discipline comes freedom

Aristotle

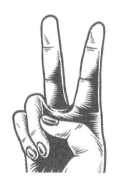

THE 2-DAY RULE TRACKER

_____

HABIT

_____

MONTH

SUN	MON	TUE	WED	THU	FRI	SAT

NOTES

_____

_____

_____

_____

THE 2-DAY RULE TRACKER

_____

HABIT

_____

MONTH

SUN	MON	TUE	WED	THU	FRI	SAT

NOTES
_____
_____
_____
_____

THE 2-DAY RULE TRACKER

HABIT

MONTH

SUN	MON	TUE	WED	THU	FRI	SAT

NOTES

THE 2-DAY RULE TRACKER

HABIT

MONTH

SUN	MON	TUE	WED	THU	FRI	SAT

NOTES

THE 2-DAY RULE TRACKER

_____

HABIT

_____

MONTH

SUN	MON	TUE	WED	THU	FRI	SAT

NOTES

_____

_____

_____

_____

Habits change into character

Ovid

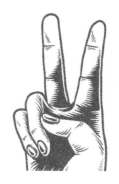

THE 2-DAY RULE TRACKER

____

HABIT

____

MONTH

SUN	MON	TUE	WED	THU	FRI	SAT

NOTES

THE 2-DAY RULE TRACKER

HABIT

MONTH

SUN	MON	TUE	WED	THU	FRI	SAT

NOTES

THE 2-DAY RULE TRACKER

_____

HABIT

_____

MONTH

SUN	MON	TUE	WED	THU	FRI	SAT

NOTES

THE 2-DAY RULE TRACKER

_____

HABIT

_____

MONTH

SUN	MON	TUE	WED	THU	FRI	SAT

NOTES

_____

_____

_____

_____

THE 2-DAY RULE TRACKER

_____

HABIT

_____

MONTH

SUN	MON	TUE	WED	THU	FRI	SAT

NOTES

_____

_____

_____

_____

Big things happen

one day at a time

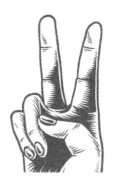

THE 2-DAY RULE TRACKER

_____

HABIT

_____

MONTH

SUN	MON	TUE	WED	THU	FRI	SAT

NOTES

_____

_____

_____

_____

THE 2-DAY RULE TRACKER

_____

HABIT

_____

MONTH

SUN	MON	TUE	WED	THU	FRI	SAT

NOTES
_____
_____
_____
_____

THE 2-DAY RULE TRACKER

_____

HABIT

_____

MONTH

SUN	MON	TUE	WED	THU	FRI	SAT

NOTES
_____
_____
_____

THE 2-DAY RULE TRACKER

HABIT

MONTH

SUN	MON	TUE	WED	THU	FRI	SAT

NOTES

THE 2-DAY RULE TRACKER

_____

HABIT

_____

MONTH

SUN	MON	TUE	WED	THU	FRI	SAT

NOTES

_____

_____

_____

_____

He is most powerful

Who has power over himself

Seneca

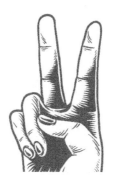

THE 2-DAY RULE TRACKER

_____

HABIT

_____

MONTH

SUN	MON	TUE	WED	THU	FRI	SAT

NOTES

_____
_____
_____
_____

THE 2-DAY RULE TRACKER

_____

HABIT

_____

MONTH

SUN	MON	TUE	WED	THU	FRI	SAT

NOTES
_____
_____
_____
_____

THE 2-DAY RULE TRACKER

———————————————————————————————

HABIT

———————————————————

MONTH

SUN	MON	TUE	WED	THU	FRI	SAT

NOTES

———————————————————————————————

———————————————————————————————

———————————————————————————————

———————————————————————————————

THE 2-DAY RULE TRACKER

HABIT

MONTH

SUN	MON	TUE	WED	THU	FRI	SAT

NOTES

THE 2-DAY RULE TRACKER

HABIT

MONTH

SUN	MON	TUE	WED	THU	FRI	SAT

NOTES

Self-control is all about moment to moment self

awareness. You catch yourself doing – or about

to do – something undesirable, see that it isn't

good for you in the long term, and as a result of

this awareness abstain from doing it.

The Ancient Sage

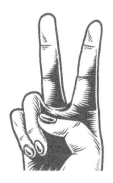

THE 2-DAY RULE TRACKER

_____

HABIT

_____

MONTH

SUN	MON	TUE	WED	THU	FRI	SAT

NOTES

_____

_____

_____

_____

THE 2-DAY RULE TRACKER

_____

HABIT

_____

MONTH

SUN	MON	TUE	WED	THU	FRI	SAT

NOTES

_____

_____

_____

_____

THE 2-DAY RULE TRACKER

HABIT

MONTH

SUN	MON	TUE	WED	THU	FRI	SAT

NOTES

THE 2-DAY RULE TRACKER

_____

HABIT

_____

MONTH

SUN	MON	TUE	WED	THU	FRI	SAT

NOTES

_____

_____

_____

_____

THE 2-DAY RULE TRACKER

_____

HABIT

_____

MONTH

SUN	MON	TUE	WED	THU	FRI	SAT

NOTES

_____

_____

_____

_____

Willpower is like a muscle

the more you train it

the stronger it gets

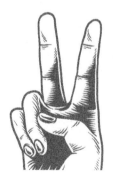

THE 2-DAY RULE TRACKER

_____

HABIT

_____

MONTH

SUN	MON	TUE	WED	THU	FRI	SAT

NOTES

_____

_____

_____

_____

THE 2-DAY RULE TRACKER

HABIT

MONTH

SUN	MON	TUE	WED	THU	FRI	SAT

NOTES

THE 2-DAY RULE TRACKER

HABIT

MONTH

SUN	MON	TUE	WED	THU	FRI	SAT

NOTES

THE 2-DAY RULE TRACKER

HABIT

MONTH

SUN	MON	TUE	WED	THU	FRI	SAT

NOTES

THE 2-DAY RULE TRACKER

SUN	MON	TUE	WED	THU	FRI	SAT

NOTES

Obstacles do not block the path.

They are the path.

Zen proverb

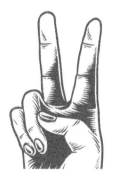

THE 2-DAY RULE TRACKER

_____

HABIT

_____

MONTH

SUN	MON	TUE	WED	THU	FRI	SAT

NOTES

_____

_____

_____

_____

THE 2-DAY RULE TRACKER

_____

HABIT

_____

MONTH

SUN	MON	TUE	WED	THU	FRI	SAT

NOTES

_____

_____

_____

_____

THE 2-DAY RULE TRACKER

HABIT

MONTH

SUN	MON	TUE	WED	THU	FRI	SAT

NOTES

THE 2-DAY RULE TRACKER

SUN	MON	TUE	WED	THU	FRI	SAT

NOTES

THE 2-DAY RULE TRACKER

HABIT

MONTH

SUN	MON	TUE	WED	THU	FRI	SAT

NOTES

If you don't change direction,

You may end up where you are heading

Lao Tzu

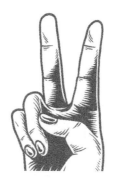

NOTES

NOTES

MONTH

MONTH

MONTH

NOTES

MONTH

MONTH

MONTH

NOTES

MONTH

MONTH

MONTH

29923324R00046